The

Pink Salt Trick

Recipe for Weight Loss

A Simple Morning Ritual for Vibrant Health and
Overall Wellness

Katharine C. Whitaker

Table of Content

Introduction

The Pink Salt Trick Unveiled

Imagine starting your day with a simple drink that promises to hydrate your body, boost your energy, and maybe even help you shed a few pounds. It's not a fancy smoothie or an expensive supplement— just a glass of warm water, a pinch of rosy-hued Himalayan pink salt, a squeeze of fresh lemon, and a touch of honey if you're feeling indulgent. This is the Pink Salt Trick, a morning ritual that's taken the wellness world by storm in 2025. If you've stumbled across this book, you're likely curious: Is this drink really a game-changer, or just another overhyped health fad? Let's dive in and find out.

What Is the Pink Salt Trick?

At its core, the Pink Salt Trick is a deceptively simple recipe: mix a quarter teaspoon of Himalayan pink salt into a glass of warm water, add a splash of lemon juice, and, if you like, stir in a teaspoon of raw honey. Sip it slowly, ideally first thing in the morning, and you're supposed to feel refreshed, energized, and ready to tackle the day. Proponents claim it does everything from improving hydration to supporting digestion, balancing hormones, and—most tantalizingly—aiding weight loss. The ingredients are affordable, the prep takes less than three minutes, and the ritual feels like a small act of self-care. But what's behind the buzz? Why has this unassuming drink captured so much attention?

The 2025 Wellness Wave

If you've scrolled through X, TikTok, or wellness blogs lately, you've probably seen the Pink Salt Trick popping up everywhere. Hashtags like #PinkSaltTrick and #MorningMagic are racking up millions of views, with influencers and everyday folks sharing their glowing reviews. Some claim they've dropped pounds, others swear by its energizing effects, and a few even whisper that celebrities like Adele might have used it as part of their wellness routines (though, spoiler alert: there's no hard evidence for that). The recipe has become a darling of the 2025 wellness culture, a time when we're all craving simple, natural solutions to feel better in a fast-paced, often overwhelming world.

This surge isn't just about the drink itself—it's part of a broader movement. After years of complex diets and pricey superfoods, people are drawn to back-to-basics health hacks. Himalayan pink salt, with its pretty pink grains and supposed mineral magic, fits the bill perfectly. It's marketed as a purer, more natural alternative to table salt, packed with trace minerals like magnesium and potassium.

Add the detoxifying allure of lemon and the soothing sweetness of honey, and you've got a recipe that feels both ancient and cutting-edge. But as with any trend, the hype comes with questions: Does it really work? And how much of the excitement is just clever marketing?

The Mission of This Book

That's where The Pink Salt Trick Recipe for Weight Loss comes in. This book isn't here to sell you a miracle or promise you'll drop 60 pounds in a month (spoiler: you won't, and anyone claiming that is probably trying to sell you something else). Instead, my goal is to give you the full picture—part guide, part myth-buster, and part cheerleader for your wellness journey. We'll explore what the Pink Salt Trick can actually do, from its potential to hydrate and energize to its role in a balanced approach to weight management. We'll dig into the science behind Himalayan pink salt, lemon, and honey, and separate fact from fiction. You'll learn how to make the drink, customize it to your tastes, and weave it into a lifestyle that supports your goals.

But more than that, this book is about empowerment. It's about taking a simple, accessible ritual and using it as a stepping stone to feel better, move more, and make choices that align with the healthiest version of you. Weight loss is part of the conversation, but it's not the whole story. The Pink Salt Trick is a tool, not a cure-all, and I'm here to show you how to use it wisely.

My 30-Day Experiment

I'll be honest—I was skeptical when I first heard about the Pink Salt Trick. Another health hacks? I'd tried enough to know that most fall short of their promises. But the simplicity intrigued me, and the ingredients were already in my kitchen. So, I decided to give it a shot for 30 days, curious to see if it lived up to the hype. Every morning, I'd mix my glass of warm water, pink salt, and lemon, sometimes adding a drizzle of honey when I needed a little sweetness. I sipped it slowly, often while journaling or watching the sunrise, turning it into a quiet moment of mindfulness.

The results? They weren't earth-shattering, but they were real. I felt more hydrated, especially on days when I'd normally reach for a second coffee. My digestion seemed smoother, and I noticed I wasn't as bloated after meals. As for weight loss, I didn't drop 20 pounds, but I did lose a couple of pounds over the month—likely because the ritual encouraged me to drink more water and make better food choices. The biggest surprise was the energy boost. I felt less sluggish in the mornings, and that motivated me to stick with my walks and yoga sessions.

My experiment wasn't perfect. Some days, the salty tang took getting used to, and I had to remind myself to keep the salt pinch small to avoid feeling thirsty later. But overall, it was a small change that made a noticeable difference. It wasn't a magic bullet, but it was a spark—a reminder that wellness doesn't have to be complicated or expensive.

Why You're Here

Maybe you picked up this book because you saw a glowing X post about the Pink Salt Trick or heard a friend raving about their morning routine. Maybe you're tired of fad diets and want something straightforward that fits your busy life. Or maybe you're just curious, wondering if this drink can really help you feel lighter, healthier, or more energized. Whatever brought you here, I'm glad you're with me.

In the pages ahead, we'll uncover the origins of the Pink Salt Trick, break down the science, and address the big question: Can it really help with weight loss? You'll get step-by-step recipes, creative variations, and practical tips to make the trick your own. We'll also talk about safety, because even simple remedies need to be used wisely. And we'll go beyond the drink, exploring how it fits into a holistic approach to wellness—think balanced meals, movement, and stress management.

This isn't about chasing quick fixes or unrealistic promises. It's about starting your day with intention, nourishing your body with purpose, and building habits that last. The Pink Salt Trick might be a small step, but small steps can lead to big changes. So, grab a glass, a pinch of pink salt, and let's get started on this journey together.

Part I
Understanding the Pink Salt Trick

The Origins and Hype

In a world overflowing with wellness trends, the Pink Salt Trick stands out for its simplicity: a pinch of Himalayan pink salt, a squeeze of lemon, a glass of warm water, and a optional drizzle of honey. This unassuming drink has sparked a frenzy in 2025, flooding social media feeds and wellness blogs with promises of hydration, energy, and even weight loss. But where did this recipe come from, and why has it captured so many imaginations? In this chapter, we'll journey through the origins of Himalayan pink salt, trace the recipe's rise to fame, unpack the celebrity rumors and marketing buzz, and explore why "simple hacks" like this one resonate so deeply in our modern health culture.

Roots of Himalayan Pink Salt

Himalayan pink salt, the star ingredient of the Pink Salt Trick, has a history that stretches back millions of years. Mined from ancient salt deposits in the Khewra Salt Mine in Pakistan's Punjab region, near the Himalayan foothills, this salt is the remnant of prehistoric oceans trapped during tectonic shifts. Its rosy hue, caused by trace minerals like iron oxide, gives it a distinctive look that's as much a visual draw as a functional one. Unlike heavily processed table salt, pink salt is hand-harvested and minimally refined, retaining its natural mineral content—a fact that wellness advocates love to highlight.

The use of pink salt in health practices isn't new. In Ayurvedic traditions, which date back over 5,000 years in India, salt has long been valued for its role in balancing the body's energies, or doshas. Ayurvedic texts, such as the Charaka Samhita, describe salt as a digestive stimulant and a carrier of minerals, often mixed with water or herbs to aid hydration and metabolism. While the Pink Salt Trick as we know it isn't explicitly mentioned in these ancient texts, the concept of salt-water solutions aligns with practices like ushapana (morning water therapy), where warm water is consumed to cleanse and prepare the body for the day.

Beyond Ayurveda, cultures worldwide have used salt for health. In traditional Chinese medicine, salt is seen as a warming, grounding substance, while in Western folk remedies, saline solutions have been used for everything from sore throats to hydration. Himalayan pink salt, with its "exotic" origins and natural appeal, has become a modern favorite, marketed as a purer alternative to table salt. Its rise in the wellness world began in the early 2000s, when health food stores started stocking it alongside goji berries and quinoa, but it wasn't until the 2020s that it found its way into viral recipes like the Pink Salt Trick.

The Rise to Fame in 2025

So, how did a simple salt-water-lemon concoction become a wellness sensation? The answer lies in the power of social media and the perfect storm of cultural trends in 2025. Platforms like X and TikTok have been instrumental in spreading the Pink Salt Trick, with hashtags like #PinkSaltTrick, #MorningRitual, and #WeightLossHack amassing millions of views. On X, users share before-and-after photos, claiming the drink helped them feel lighter or more energized, while TikTok videos show aesthetically pleasing shots of pink salt dissolving in golden morning light, often set to soothing music.

Wellness blogs have also played a big role. Sites like Cook up Taste and My Tasty Curry have published detailed guides on the recipe, complete with user comments praising its simplicity and taste. These blogs often frame the Pink Salt Trick as a "Magic Morning Mix" or "sole water" (a term borrowed from older wellness practices, referring to a saturated salt-water solution). The recipe's accessibility—cheap ingredients, minimal prep time—makes it easy for anyone to try, fueling its viral spread.

The timing couldn't be better. In 2025, we're seeing a backlash against overly complex health trends. After years of keto diets, intermittent fasting, and $50 superfood powders, people are craving straightforward solutions. The Pink Salt Trick fits this mood perfectly: it's affordable (a bag of pink salt costs less than $10), requires no special equipment, and feels like a ritual you can actually stick to. Posts on X often describe it as "the one health hack I can do every day," reflecting a collective desire for wellness that doesn't feel like a second job.

Celebrity Connections and Marketing Claims

No wellness trend is complete without a sprinkle of celebrity sparkle, and the Pink Salt Trick is no exception. Rumors have swirled that stars like Adele, known for her dramatic weight loss journey, might have used the Pink Salt Trick as part of their regimens. These claims, often amplified by clickbait ads and shady websites, suggest the drink is a secret weapon for shedding pounds fast. One X post from early 2025 speculated, "Is this what Adele's been sipping? #PinkSaltTrick," sparking thousands of retweets before fading into the digital ether.

Let's be clear: there's no evidence linking Adele or any celebrity to the Pink Salt Trick. These rumors are likely the work of savvy marketers who know that tying a product to a famous name boosts its allure. As MalwareTips Blog (2024) points out, some online ads for the Pink Salt Trick use fake endorsements and exaggerated claims—like losing 60 pounds in weeks without diet or exercise—to lure clicks. These tactics are part of a broader pattern in wellness marketing, where simple remedies are hyped as miracles to sell supplements or e-books.

That said, the celebrity buzz isn't entirely baseless. High-profile figures often embrace hydration-focused rituals, and pink salt has popped up in celebrity wellness routines, from salt lamps to cooking. Gwyneth Paltrow's Goop, for instance, has praised Himalayan salt for its "vibrational energy" (a claim we'll politely sidestep). The Pink Salt Trick's association with these trends gives it a glamorous sheen, even if the reality is more grounded.

The Allure of Simple Hacks

Why has the Pink Salt Trick struck such a chord? It's not just about pink salt or social media—it's about the broader appeal of "simple hacks" in our health-obsessed culture. In 2025, we're bombarded with information overload: one day, a study says coffee is a superfood; the next, it's a health risk. Diets come and go, each promising transformation but often delivering frustration. Against this backdrop, the Pink Salt Trick feels like a breath of fresh air.

The recipe taps into several psychological and cultural trends:

- Simplicity: With just four ingredients and three minutes of prep, it's a low-barrier entry to wellness. No blenders, no meal plans, no gym membership required.

- Ritual: Drinking it in the morning becomes a moment of self-care, like lighting a candle or writing in a journal. It's less about the drink and more about the intention behind it.

- Nostalgia: The idea of salt and lemon harks back to traditional remedies, evoking a sense of timeless wisdom in a tech-driven world.

- Community: Social media creates a shared experience, with users posting their variations (ginger-infused, minty twists) and cheering each other on.

This allure is amplified by the wellness industry's knack for storytelling. Himalayan pink salt isn't just salt—it's "ancient," "pristine," "from the heart of the Himalayas." Never mind that it's mined in Pakistan, not the actual Himalayas; the narrative is compelling. Add lemon's "detox" aura and honey's "natural sweetness," and you've got a recipe that feels like it's been whispered down through generations, even if its current form is a 21st-century invention.

Navigating the Hype

The Pink Salt Trick's rise is a testament to the power of community, storytelling, and the human desire for health solutions that feel within reach. Its roots in Ayurvedic and traditional practices give it a foundation, but its 2025 popularity is pure modern magic—social media, marketing, and a cultural craving for simplicity. The celebrity rumors and weight loss claims add fuel to the fire, but they also invite skepticism, which we'll tackle in the next chapter.

As you read on, keep this in mind: the Pink Salt Trick is neither a miracle nor a scam. It's a tool, one that can hydrate, energize, and inspire when used thoughtfully. By understanding its origins and the hype that surrounds it, you're better equipped to sip with purpose, not just follow the crowd. Let's move forward and dive into the science behind this drink, separating fact from fiction to uncover what it can really do for you.

The Science Behind the Ingredients

The Pink Salt Trick is more than just a trendy drink—it's a blend of ingredients that each bring something to the table. Himalayan pink salt, lemon juice, warm water, and optional honey work together to create a ritual that feels refreshing and purposeful. But what does science say about these components? Are they really as powerful as the wellness world claims, or is this just a case of clever marketing? In this chapter, we'll dive into the research behind each ingredient, exploring their benefits, limitations, and how they contribute to the Pink Salt Trick's appeal. From hydration to digestion, let's unpack what's really going on in your glass.

Himalayan Pink Salt: The Star of the Show

Himalayan pink salt is the heart of the Pink Salt Trick, prized for its rosy hue and supposed mineral richness. Unlike regular table salt, which is heavily processed, pink salt is mined from ancient salt deposits in the Punjab region of Pakistan, near the Himalayan foothills. Its pink color comes from trace minerals like iron oxide, and it's often marketed as a "natural" alternative packed with health benefits. But what does the science say?

Trace Minerals: Fact or Hype?

Himalayan pink salt contains up to 84 trace minerals, including magnesium, potassium, calcium, and iron, which sound impressive on paper. These minerals are essential for bodily functions—magnesium supports muscle relaxation, potassium helps regulate fluid balance, and iron aids oxygen transport. Wellness blogs often claim these minerals make pink salt a nutritional powerhouse compared to table salt.

However, the reality is less glamorous. According to Healthline (2023), while pink salt does contain these minerals, the amounts are so small that they're unlikely to significantly impact your health. For example, a quarter teaspoon of pink salt—the amount used in the Pink Salt Trick—provides less than 1% of your daily magnesium or potassium needs. You'd need to consume impractically large amounts to get meaningful doses, which would bring its own risks due to sodium content. So, while the minerals add a nice story, they're not the main reason to sip this drink.

Hydration: The Real Benefit

Where pink salt shines is in its role as an electrolyte. Sodium, the primary component of all salt, helps your body retain water, which is crucial for hydration. When you drink the Pink Salt Trick, the small amount of sodium in the salt can enhance water absorption, making you feel more hydrated than plain water alone.

This is why athletes often turn to electrolyte drinks after intense workouts. A 2016 study in the Journal of the International Society of Sports Nutrition found that low doses of sodium in water improve hydration markers, especially in dehydrated individuals.

For the average person, this hydration boost can translate to feeling more alert and less sluggish, especially in the morning. However, the Pink Salt Trick isn't a sports drink—it's a gentle, daily ritual, and its hydration benefits are modest but noticeable, particularly if you're prone to skipping water or feeling parched after sleep.

Sodium Risks: A Word of Caution

The flip side of sodium is its potential risks. Too much salt can raise blood pressure, strain kidneys, and lead to water retention, which is the opposite of what you want if you're aiming for weight loss. The American Heart Association recommends no more than 2,300 mg of sodium daily (about 1 teaspoon of salt), with an ideal limit of 1,500 mg for most adults. A quarter teaspoon of Himalayan pink salt contains roughly 400–500 mg of sodium, which is safe for most people as part of the Pink Salt Trick, but it's not something to overdo.

WebMD (2022) warns that individuals with hypertension, kidney disease, or heart conditions should be cautious with any added salt, including pink salt. If you're sensitive to sodium or on a low-sodium diet, consult your doctor before making this drink a daily habit. The key is moderation—stick to the recommended pinch and avoid piling on salty foods elsewhere in your day.

Lemon Juice: A Zesty Boost

Lemon juice is the second pillar of the Pink Salt Trick, adding a bright, tangy flavor and a host of health benefits. Squeezing half a teaspoon of fresh lemon juice (about a quarter of a lemon) into your drink doesn't just make it taste better—it brings some science-backed perks to the mix.

Vitamin C and Antioxidants

Lemons are rich in vitamin C, a powerful antioxidant that supports immune health, skin repair, and tissue maintenance. A 2020 article in Medical News Today notes that even small amounts of lemon juice contribute to your daily vitamin C needs, which is about 75-90 mg for adults. The half teaspoon in the Pink Salt Trick provides a modest dose—roughly 2-3 mg—but it's a nice bonus, especially if you're sipping it daily.

Antioxidants in lemon juice, including flavonoids, help combat oxidative stress in the body, which is linked to aging and chronic diseases. While the amount in the Pink Salt Trick is small, it's part of a cumulative effect if you're eating other antioxidant-rich foods like berries or greens.

Digestion Benefits

Lemon juice is often praised for kickstarting digestion, and there's some truth to this. The citric acid in lemons may stimulate saliva and gastric juices, preparing your stomach for food. A 2019 study in Food Science & Nutrition found that citrus compounds can enhance digestive enzyme activity, potentially easing bloating or sluggishness. For many, the Pink Salt Trick's lemon component feels like a gentle wake-up call for the gut, especially when taken on an empty stomach.

That said, the "detox" claims surrounding lemon juice are overstated. Your liver and kidneys already handle detoxification, and no single food or drink can "cleanse" your system. Instead, think of lemon juice as a supportive player, aiding digestion and adding a refreshing zing that makes the drink more enjoyable.

Considerations

Fresh lemon juice is best for maximum flavor and nutrients, but bottled juice can work in a pinch (just check for added sugars or preservatives). Be mindful of lemon's acidity, which can erode tooth enamel over time. Sipping through a straw or rinsing your mouth with water afterward can protect your teeth.

Honey: The Optional Sweetener

Honey is an optional ingredient in the Pink Salt Trick, but it's a popular addition for those who find the salty-lemon combo a bit tart. A teaspoon of raw honey adds a touch of sweetness and its own set of health properties, but it also comes with caveats.

Antioxidants and Natural Benefits

Raw honey is more than just a sweetener—it's a natural source of antioxidants, including polyphenols, which may reduce inflammation and protect against chronic diseases. A 2021 review in Antioxidants highlighted honey's potential to support heart health and improve cholesterol levels when used in moderation. Raw, unprocessed honey also contains trace enzymes and pollen that may offer minor immune benefits, though these are diminished in pasteurized varieties.

In the Pink Salt Trick, a teaspoon of honey adds a subtle flavor boost, making the drink more palatable for beginners. It also provides a quick energy source, as honey is primarily simple sugars (glucose and fructose), which your body absorbs rapidly.

Calorie Considerations

The downside? Honey is calorie-dense, with about 20-22 calories per teaspoon. If you're aiming for weight loss, this might seem counterintuitive, especially since the Pink Salt Trick is often marketed as a slimming aid. However, one teaspoon is a small amount, and its calories are unlikely to derail your goals if you're mindful of your overall diet. For those watching sugar intake, especially if you have diabetes, you might skip honey or use a sugar-free alternative like stevia, though this changes the flavor profile.

Healthline (2023) advises choosing raw, organic honey for maximum benefits, as processed honey often lacks antioxidants and may contain added sugars. If you include honey, use it sparingly and treat it as a treat, not a health food.

Warm Water: The Unsung Hero

Warm water might seem like the least exciting part of the Pink Salt Trick, but it's the foundation that ties everything together. The temperature of the water—ideally lukewarm, around 98-105°F (37-40°C)—plays a surprising role in the drink's effectiveness.

Why Temperature Matters

Warm water is easier for your body to absorb than cold water, as it's closer to your internal body temperature. A 2018 study in The Journal of Physiology found that lukewarm fluids pass through the stomach faster than cold ones, promoting quicker hydration and digestion. This is why many traditional practices, like Ayurveda, recommend warm water in the morning to "wake up" the digestive system.

For the Pink Salt Trick, warm water helps dissolve the pink salt fully, ensuring the sodium and minerals are evenly distributed. It also enhances the lemon's flavor and makes the drink feel soothing, like a gentle hug for your insides. Cold water can work, but it may slow digestion slightly and feel less comforting, especially in cooler months.

Practical Tips

Use filtered water to avoid impurities, and aim for a temperature that's warm but not scalding—think "pleasant to sip," not "boiling tea." If you're new to warm water drinks, it might take a day or two to adjust, but most people find it grows on them.

Comparison with Regular Salt and Electrolyte Drinks

How does Himalayan pink salt stack up against regular table salt or popular electrolyte drinks like Gatorade? Let's break it down.

Pink Salt vs. Table Salt

Table salt is typically processed to remove impurities and minerals, leaving mostly sodium chloride. It's often fortified with iodine to prevent deficiency, a feature pink salt lacks.

Pink salt, by contrast, retains trace minerals and has slightly less sodium per gram due to its coarser structure. A 2022 WebMD article notes that pink salt's mineral content is negligible for health, but its lower processing appeals to those seeking "natural" options.

In the Pink Salt Trick, pink salt's subtle flavor and visual appeal make it more inviting than table salt, which can taste harsher. However, both provide sodium for hydration, so table salt could technically work in a pinch (though you'd miss the pink salt's mystique). If you use table salt, ensure it's non-iodized to avoid an off taste, and be aware of iodine needs elsewhere in your diet.

Pink Salt vs. Electrolyte Drinks

Commercial electrolyte drinks like Gatorade or Pedialyte are designed for rapid rehydration, often after intense exercise or illness. They contain sodium, potassium, and sugars in precise ratios, backed by decades of research. The Pink Salt Trick, with its small sodium dose and lemon's potassium, mimics a very mild electrolyte drink but lacks the concentrated punch of these products.

A key difference is sugar content. Electrolyte drinks often have added sugars or artificial sweeteners, which can add calories or cause digestive issues for some. The Pink Salt Trick, especially without honey, is lower in calories and free of artificial additives, making it a cleaner option for daily use. However, it's not a replacement for medical-grade rehydration in cases of severe dehydration—stick to doctor-recommended solutions for that.

What the Studies Say

The science on the Pink Salt Trick's ingredients is a mix of promising and sobering. Here's a summary of key findings from credible sources:

- Himalayan Pink Salt: Medical News Today (2021) states there's no evidence pink salt is superior to table salt for health outcomes. Its trace minerals are present in such small amounts that they don't significantly contribute to nutrition. However, its sodium content supports hydration, as confirmed by studies like the one in Journal of the International Society of Sports Nutrition (2016).

- Lemon Juice: Research in Food Science & Nutrition (2019) supports lemon's role in stimulating digestion, but Healthline (2023) debunks detox claims, noting that vitamin C and antioxidants are the primary benefits.

- Honey: A 2021 Antioxidants review highlights honey's anti-inflammatory potential, but its high calorie content requires moderation, as per WebMD (2022).

- Warm Water: The Journal of Physiology (2018) confirms warm water's faster absorption, supporting its use in morning rituals.

The Pink Salt Trick's benefits—hydration, mild digestive support, and a slight energy boost—are real but modest. Claims of dramatic weight loss or miraculous health transformations lack evidence and should be approached with skepticism. The drink's power lies in its simplicity and synergy, not in any single ingredient being a magic bullet.

So, what does this mean for your morning glass of Pink Salt Trick? The science tells us it's a solid choice for hydration and digestion, thanks to pink salt's sodium, lemon's citric acid, and warm water's absorbability. Honey adds a touch of sweetness and antioxidants, but it's optional for those watching calories. While the trace minerals in pink salt make for a compelling story, they're not the star players—sodium and hydration are.

This drink isn't going to melt pounds or cure ailments, but it can be a refreshing, intentional start to your day. By understanding the science, you can approach the Pink Salt Trick with realistic expectations, appreciating what it does well without falling for exaggerated hype. In the next chapter, we'll tackle those myths head-on, separating fact from fiction to ensure you're sipping with confidence.

The Pink Salt Trick has a certain magic to it—a simple drink that feels like a secret weapon for better health. But with its rise to fame in 2025, it's also been swept up in a tide of hype, with some claims stretching far beyond what a glass of salty lemon water can deliver. Promises of losing 60 pounds in weeks or curing every ailment under the sun have flooded the internet, leaving many wondering: Is this too good to be true? Spoiler alert: Yes, it often is. In this chapter, we'll separate fact from fiction, debunk the biggest myths, expose marketing scams, and set realistic expectations for what the Pink Salt Trick can—and can't—do. Let's clear the air and focus on how this drink can genuinely support your wellness journey.

Common Myths: Sorting Hype from Reality

The Pink Salt Trick's popularity has made it a magnet for exaggerated claims, especially on social media and shady websites. Here are some of the most common myths circulating in 2025, along with the truth behind them:

Myth 1: "Lose 60 Pounds in Weeks!"

Perhaps the most alluring claim is that the Pink Salt Trick can melt away massive amounts of weight in record time. Ads on X and pop-up websites proclaim, "Drop 60 pounds in 6 weeks with this one simple trick!" accompanied by dramatic before-and-after photos. The idea that a daily glass of salt water could lead to such results is tempting, but it's not grounded in science.

The reality? Weight loss requires a calorie deficit—burning more calories than you consume through a combination of diet, exercise, and lifestyle changes. The Pink Salt Trick, while hydrating and refreshing, doesn't directly burn fat or alter your metabolism. A 2024 analysis by MalwareTips Blog debunked these claims, noting that such promises are biologically implausible without extreme dietary restrictions or other interventions. If you see a 60-pound weight loss story tied to this drink, it's likely fabricated or paired with undisclosed changes like crash dieting.

Myth 2: "Cures All Ailments"

Another pervasive myth is that the Pink Salt Trick is a cure-all, capable of fixing everything from chronic fatigue to hormonal imbalances to serious illnesses. Some wellness influencers on TikTok have called it a "detox elixir" that "flushes toxins" or "resets your body." Others claim it can balance pH levels, cure migraines, or even prevent disease.

The truth is far less dramatic. As Medical News Today (2021) explains, the human body already has robust systems—your liver, kidneys, and lungs—for detoxification, and no single drink can "reset" them. Himalayan pink salt provides sodium and trace minerals, but these are present in tiny amounts that don't significantly impact chronic conditions. Lemon juice offers vitamin C and may aid digestion, but it's not a cure for migraines or hormonal issues. Claims about pH balance are also misleading; your body tightly regulates its pH, and diet has minimal effect, per Healthline (2023). While the Pink Salt Trick can make you feel refreshed, it's not a medical miracle.

Myth 3: "It's a Magic Bullet for Everyone"

Some proponents suggest the Pink Salt Trick is universally beneficial, suitable for all ages, health conditions, and lifestyles. Posts on X often tout it as "the one hack everyone needs," implying it's a one-size-fits-all solution.

In reality, the drink isn't for everyone. People with hypertension, kidney disease, or sodium sensitivities should approach it cautiously, as even a small amount of salt can exacerbate these conditions, according to WebMD (2022). Pregnant women and those on certain medications (like diuretics) also need medical guidance before adding extra sodium. The Pink Salt Trick is a tool, not a universal fix, and its benefits depend on your individual health and how you use it.

The Truth About Weight Loss

With the weight loss hype debunked, you might be wondering: Does the Pink Salt Trick have any role in weight management? The answer is yes, but it's indirect and far more modest than the ads suggest. Let's break down how it might contribute and why it's not a standalone solution.

No Direct Mechanism

The Pink Salt Trick doesn't directly cause weight loss. Its core ingredients—Himalayan pink salt, lemon juice, warm water, and optional honey—don't contain compounds that burn fat or boost metabolism significantly. Sodium aids hydration, lemon supports digestion, and honey provides a small energy boost, but none of these directly translate to shedding pounds. A 2023 Quora discussion on pink salt and weight loss echoed this, with experts noting that any weight loss from such drinks is likely due to water weight or placebo-driven behavior changes, not the drink itself.

Indirect Benefits

That said, the Pink Salt Trick can support weight management indirectly by fostering habits that align with a healthy lifestyle:

- Better Hydration: Sodium in pink salt helps your body retain water, improving hydration. A 2016 study in the Journal of the International Society of Sports Nutrition found that proper hydration can reduce perceived hunger and prevent overeating, as thirst is often mistaken for hunger. Starting your day with the Pink Salt Trick might keep you sipping water, subtly curbing unnecessary snacking.

- Reduced Cravings: The drink's tangy, slightly salty flavor can satisfy taste buds, potentially reducing cravings for sugary or processed foods. Some users report that it helps them skip morning pastries in favor of healthier breakfasts, an anecdotal benefit that aligns with mindful eating principles.

- Energy for Activity: Feeling hydrated and refreshed can boost your energy, making you more likely to stick with exercise or daily movement. A small 2019 study in Appetite suggested that improved hydration enhances mood and motivation, which can support active lifestyles.

- Mindful Ritual: The act of preparing and sipping the drink creates a moment of intention, encouraging mindfulness. This can spill over into other choices, like opting for a balanced lunch or prioritizing sleep, both critical for weight management.

These benefits are real but subtle. For example, losing a couple of pounds over a month might happen if the Pink Salt Trick helps you drink more water, eat less junk food, and move more—but it's the broader lifestyle changes driving the results, not the drink alone.

The Catch

Any weight loss tied to the Pink Salt Trick requires consistency and context. If you're sipping it while eating high-calorie foods or skipping exercise, don't expect results. Honey, if used, adds calories (about 20 per teaspoon), which can accumulate if you're not mindful. And overusing salt can lead to water retention, making you feel bloated rather than lighter. The key is to see the Pink Salt Trick as a supportive habit, not a magic potion.

Marketing Scams and Red Flags

The Pink Salt Trick's popularity has made it a target for unscrupulous marketers, and 2025 is no stranger to wellness scams. Understanding these red flags can help you navigate the hype and protect your wallet and health.

Fake Endorsements

One common tactic is fake celebrity endorsements. As mentioned in Chapter 1, rumors about Adele or other stars using the Pink Salt Trick are unverified and often fabricated. Malware Tips Blog (2024) exposed ads that use doctored images or quotes to link celebrities to the drink, driving clicks to dubious websites. These sites may push expensive "Pink Salt Trick supplements" or subscriptions, claiming they're the "real" formula. Stick to the simple recipe in this book—there's no need for costly add-ons.

High-Pressure Ads

Another red flag is high-pressure marketing. Ads with countdown timers ("Only 3 bottles left!") or urgent language ("Lose weight NOW or regret it!") are designed to trigger impulse buys. Legitimate health advice doesn't rely on fear or scarcity. If an ad feels pushy or too good to be true, it probably is.

Unrealistic Promises

Claims like "Lose 60 pounds without diet or exercise" are a hallmark of scams. Healthline (2023) warns that sustainable weight loss typically occurs at a rate of 0.5–2 pounds per week, requiring a calorie deficit of 500–1,000 calories daily. Any product or hack promising rapid, effortless results is likely overselling. Check the fine print—many of these ads admit that results "require diet and exercise," undermining their own claims.

How to Spot Legit Advice

To avoid scams, stick to credible sources like peer-reviewed studies, reputable health sites (e.g., WebMD, Medical News Today), or books like this one that prioritize transparency. On X, look for user reviews from real people sharing balanced experiences, not bots or paid influencers. If you're buying pink salt, choose food-grade brands from trusted retailers, not overpriced "miracle blends" online.

Realistic Goals: What the Pink Salt Trick Can Do

Now that we've cleared away the myths and scams, let's focus on what the Pink Salt Trick can offer. When used as part of a broader lifestyle, it can be a valuable tool for wellness, with benefits that are modest but meaningful. Here's what you can realistically expect:

Improved Energy

The hydration boost from pink salt and warm water can help you feel more alert, especially in the morning. Many users report a subtle lift in energy, like swapping a sluggish start for a brighter one. This isn't a caffeine-level jolt but a gentle nudge that can motivate you to tackle your day, whether that's a workout or a busy work schedule.

Better Digestion

Lemon juice's citric acid may stimulate digestive juices, easing bloating or sluggishness, as noted in a 2019 Food Science & Nutrition study. The warm water helps, too, moving things along in your gut. If you often feel heavy after meals, the Pink Salt Trick might make mornings feel lighter, setting a positive tone for eating mindfully.

Enhanced Wellness

The ritual of preparing and sipping the drink fosters mindfulness, a cornerstone of wellness. It's a moment to pause, breathe, and prioritize your health, which can ripple into other habits—choosing a salad over fries, walking instead of scrolling, or getting to bed earlier. Over time, these small choices add up, supporting overall health and potentially weight management.

A Starting Point for Weight Management

While the Pink Salt Trick won't directly burn fat, it can be a catalyst for healthier habits. By keeping you hydrated, reducing cravings, and boosting energy, it might help you stick to a balanced diet and active routine. For example, a reader shared on X: "The Pink Salt Trick didn't make me skinny, but it got me drinking water and eating better—down 5 pounds in a month!" This kind of gradual progress is realistic and sustainable.

What It's Not

The Pink Salt Trick isn't a quick fix or a substitute for professional medical advice. It won't cure chronic conditions, replace a nutrient-rich diet, or make up for a sedentary lifestyle. If weight loss is your goal, pair it with a calorie-conscious diet, regular movement, and stress management, as we'll explore in later chapters.

Moving Forward with Clarity

The Pink Salt Trick is a simple, accessible ritual with real benefits, but it's not a miracle worker. By debunking myths like "lose 60 pounds in weeks" or "cures all ailments," we can approach it with clear eyes, appreciating its role in hydration, digestion, and mindfulness without expecting the impossible. The marketing scams are a reminder to stay savvy—trust your instincts, avoid flashy promises, and focus on credible advice.

As you sip your Pink Salt Trick, think of it as a small, intentional step toward wellness. It's not about transforming your body overnight but about building habits that make you feel good inside and out. In the next chapter, we'll get practical, diving into the core recipe and creative variations to make this drink your own. With realistic expectations in place, you're ready to harness the Pink Salt Trick for what it truly offers—a refreshing start to a healthier you.

Part II:

The Pink Salt Trick in

Practice

The Core Recipe and Variations

Now that we've explored the origins, science, and realistic expectations of the Pink Salt Trick, it's time to roll up your sleeves and make it! This chapter is your go-to guide for preparing the classic Pink Salt Trick recipe, complete with step-by-step instructions and practical tips to ensure success. But why stop at the basics? We'll also dive into creative variations to keep things fresh, from a zesty ginger boost to a cooling mint twist. Plus, you'll find advice on sourcing quality ingredients, the tools you'll need, and how to streamline prep for busy mornings. Whether you're a wellness newbie or a seasoned health enthusiast, this chapter will help you make the Pink Salt Trick your own.

The Classic Pink Salt Trick Recipe

The beauty of the Pink Salt Trick lies in its simplicity: four ingredients, three minutes, and a glass of refreshing goodness. The classic recipe is designed to hydrate, energize, and kickstart your day, with a balance of salty, tangy, and subtly sweet flavors. Here's everything you need to know to whip it up.

Ingredients (Serves 1)

- Warm Water: 8–12 oz (1–1.5 cups), filtered, heated to 98–105°F (37–40°C).

- Himalayan Pink Salt: 1/4 tsp, finely ground, food-grade.

- Fresh Lemon Juice: 1/2 tsp (about 1/4 of a small lemon, freshly squeezed).

- Raw Honey (optional): 1 tsp, preferably organic and unprocessed.

Step-by-Step Guide

- Heat the Water: Pour 8–12 oz of filtered water into a small pot or kettle and warm it to a comfortable sipping temperature (lukewarm, not boiling). Alternatively, heat water in a microwave-safe glass for 20–30 seconds, checking to avoid overheating. Aim for a temperature that feels soothing, like a warm hug for your stomach.

- Add the Pink Salt: Measure 1/4 tsp of finely ground Himalayan pink salt and stir it into the warm water until fully dissolved. This usually takes 10–15 seconds. If the salt doesn't dissolve completely, your water may be too cool—warm it slightly more.

- Squeeze the Lemon: Cut a fresh lemon into quarters and squeeze about 1/2 tsp of juice (roughly 1/4 of the lemon) into the water. Stir gently to mix. For best flavor and nutrients, use fresh lemons rather than bottled juice, which may contain preservatives or lose potency over time.

- Optional Honey: If you prefer a touch of sweetness, add 1 tsp of raw honey and stir until it melts into the drink. Honey softens the salty-tangy edge, but skip it if you're watching calories or prefer a sharper flavor.

- Sip Slowly: Pour the drink into a favorite glass or mug and sip it slowly, ideally on an empty stomach in the morning. Take your time to savor the ritual—think of it as a moment of mindfulness to start your day.

Tips for Success

- Use Food-Grade Salt: Ensure your Himalayan pink salt is labeled food-grade, as some pink salt is sold for baths or lamps and may contain impurities. Finely ground salt dissolves better than coarse grains.

- Sip Through a Straw: Lemon's acidity can wear on tooth enamel over time. Using a straw minimizes contact with teeth, and rinsing your mouth with plain water afterward helps, too.

- Adjust to Taste: If the drink feels too salty or tart, tweak the ratios slightly (e.g., reduce salt to 1/8 tsp or add a splash more water). It may take a few tries to find your perfect balance.

- Make It a Ritual: Pair the drink with a morning habit, like stretching, journaling, or watching the sunrise, to anchor it in your routine. This boosts the feel-good factor and makes it easier to stick with.

- Stay Consistent: For benefits like hydration and digestion, sip the Pink Salt Trick daily, but stick to one serving to avoid excess sodium (more on safety in Chapter 6).

Prep Time

- Total Time: 2–3 minutes (1 minute to heat water, 1–2 minutes to mix).

Creative Variations to Spice It Up

The classic Pink Salt Trick is a solid foundation, but variety keeps things exciting. These variations let you customize the drink to your taste, health goals, or mood, while maintaining its core benefits. Whether you want a digestive boost, a cooling twist, or a low-calorie option, there's a version for you. Below are four delicious spins to try.

Ginger Boost: For Digestion

- Why It Works: Ginger is a superstar for digestion, with compounds like gingerol that soothe the stomach and reduce bloating, per a 2019 study in Food Science & Nutrition. It adds a spicy warmth that complements the salt and lemon.

- Ingredients:

  - Classic recipe (8–12 oz warm water, 1/4 tsp pink salt, 1/2 tsp lemon juice, optional 1 tsp honey).

  - 1/4 tsp freshly grated ginger (or 1/8 tsp ground ginger in a pinch).

- Instructions: Add the grated ginger to the warm water along with the pink salt, stirring until both dissolve. Follow with lemon juice and honey, if using. Strain if you prefer a smoother texture, or leave the ginger bits for extra zing.

- Tip: Start with a small amount of ginger to avoid overpowering the drink. This variation is great for mornings when you feel sluggish or after a heavy meal the night before.

Mint Refresh: For a Cooling Twist

- Why It Works: Fresh mint adds a cooling, refreshing note that balances the salt's intensity, making the drink feel like a spa-inspired treat. Mint may also ease digestion, according to Healthline (2023).

- Ingredients:

  - Classic recipe (8–12 oz warm water, 1/4 tsp pink salt, 1/2 tsp lemon juice, optional 1 tsp honey).

  - 2–3 fresh mint leaves, gently crushed.

- Instructions: After dissolving the pink salt in warm water, add the crushed mint leaves and let them steep for 1–2 minutes. Stir in lemon juice and honey, if desired, and sip through a straw for a crisp, invigorating experience.

- Tip: Crush the mint gently between your fingers to release its oils without breaking it into bits. This variation is perfect for warm days or when you want a lighter, fresher flavor.

Coconut Electrolyte: For Extra Hydration

- Why It Works: Coconut water is naturally rich in potassium and electrolytes, enhancing the drink's hydration power. It's a great choice for active days or post-workout recovery, as noted in a 2018 Journal of the International Society of Sports Nutrition study.

- Ingredients:

    - 6 oz warm water, 1/4 tsp pink salt, 1/2 tsp lemon juice, optional 1 tsp honey.

    - 4 oz unsweetened coconut water (pure, no added sugars).

- Instructions: Combine warm water and coconut water, then dissolve the pink salt. Add lemon juice and honey, if using, and stir well. The coconut water adds a subtle sweetness, so you may not need honey.

- Tip: Choose 100% pure coconut water, not flavored or sweetened versions, to keep calories low. Sip this after exercise or on hot days for a natural electrolyte boost.

Sugar-Free: For Low-Calorie Goals

- Why It Works: Skipping honey reduces the drink's calorie count, making it ideal for those focused-on weight management or monitoring sugar intake, especially for diabetes management.

- Ingredients:

    - Classic recipe (8–12 oz warm water, 1/4 tsp pink salt, 1/2 tsp lemon juice).

    - No honey or sweeteners.

- Instructions: Follow the classic recipe, omitting the honey. If the flavor feels too sharp, increase the water to 12 oz or reduce the lemon juice to 1/4 tsp for a milder taste.

- Tip: Embrace the tangy-salt profile as a palate cleanser. This version is perfect for those who want the Pink Salt Trick's benefits without any added calories.

Tools and Sourcing: Getting It Right

To make the Pink Salt Trick consistently delicious, you'll need a few basic tools and high-quality ingredients. Here's what you need and where to find it.

Tools

- Glass or Mug: A 12–16 oz glass or ceramic mug works best for sipping. Choose one you love to make the ritual special.

- Measuring Spoons: Precise measurements (1/4 tsp for salt, 1/2 tsp for lemon juice, 1 tsp for honey) ensure the right balance.

- Small Pot or Kettle: For heating water. A microwave-safe glass works for quick prep, but a kettle offers better temperature control.

- Citrus Juicer or Fork: A handheld juicer makes squeezing lemons easy, but you can use a fork to extract juice from a lemon quarter.

- Grater (Optional): For the ginger variation, a microplane or fine grater creates perfect ginger shreds.

- Straw (Recommended): A reusable silicone or stainless steel straw protects your teeth from lemon's acidity.

Sourcing Quality Ingredients

- Himalayan Pink Salt: Look for food-grade, finely ground pink salt from reputable brands like Morton, McCormick, or Thrive Market. Avoid "decorative" or "bath" salts, which aren't safe for consumption. Check labels for purity—no additives or anti-caking agents. Available at grocery stores, health food shops, or online retailers like Amazon or iHerb (prices range from $5–$10 for a 1-lb bag).

- Lemons: Opt for fresh, organic lemons for maximum flavor and no pesticide residue. Farmers' markets, Whole Foods, or local grocers are great sources. Choose firm, bright yellow lemons with thin skins for juiciness. If organic isn't available, wash thoroughly.

- Raw Honey: Select raw, unprocessed honey for antioxidants and flavor. Brands like Nature Nate's or local apiaries are ideal. Find it at health food stores, co-ops, or online. Look for "100% pure" or "raw" on the label to avoid processed blends (about $8–$15 for a 16-oz jar).

- Coconut Water and Extras: For variations, choose pure, unsweetened coconut water (e.g., Vita Coco, Harmless Harvest) from grocery stores. Fresh mint and ginger are widely available in produce sections or can be grown at home for freshness.

Budget Tip

The Pink Salt Trick is wallet-friendly. A 1-lb bag of pink salt makes over 900 servings, lemons cost pennies each, and a jar of honey lasts months. Shop in bulk or at discount stores like Trader Joe's or Costco to save more.

Prep Time, Storage, and Batch-Making

The Pink Salt Trick is designed for daily ease, but a little planning can make it even simpler, especially for busy mornings.

Prep Time

- Single Serving: 2–3 minutes, including heating water and mixing.

- With Variations: Add 1–2 minutes for grating ginger or crushing mint.

Storage Tips

- Fresh Is Best: The drink is most effective when made fresh, as lemon juice loses vitamin C potency over time, and dissolved salt can taste flat if stored.

- Prepped Ingredients: You can pre-squeeze lemon juice and store it in an airtight container in the fridge for up to 2 days, but fresh-squeezed is ideal. Ginger can be grated and frozen in small portions for quick use. Mint leaves stay fresh in a damp paper towel in the fridge for 3–5 days.

- Honey and Salt: Store pink salt in a cool, dry place (it lasts indefinitely). Keep honey in a sealed jar at room temperature to prevent crystallization.

Batch-Making Advice

While daily prep is recommended for freshness, you can streamline the process for convenience:

- Pre-Measure Salt: Portion 1/4 tsp servings of pink salt into small containers or bags for a week's worth of drinks. Store in a dry, airtight container.

- Lemon Prep: Squeeze several lemons at once and store the juice in a glass jar in the fridge. Use within 2 days for best flavor.

- Morning Setup: Set out your glass, measuring spoons, and ingredients the night before to save time.

- Batch for Travel: If you're on the go, mix a dry blend of 1/4 tsp pink salt and a pinch of dried lemon powder (available at health stores) in a small packet. Add to warm water and stir when ready. Note: This lacks fresh lemon's vibrancy but works in a pinch.

Caution

Don't pre-mix large batches of the full drink (water, salt, lemon, honey) and store them, as the flavor degrades, and there's a risk of bacterial growth, especially with honey or lemon. Make only what you'll sip immediately.

Making It Your Own

The Pink Salt Trick is more than a recipe—it's a canvas for creativity and self-care. The classic version is a fantastic starting point, offering hydration and a gentle digestive boost in just a few sips. But the variations let you tailor it to your needs, whether you're craving a spicy kick, a cooling vibe, or a calorie-free option. As you experiment, pay attention to how your body feels. Does the ginger version settle your stomach? Does mint make mornings feel brighter? These small tweaks can turn a routine into a ritual you look forward to.

With quality ingredients, a few simple tools, and a minute or two each morning, you're ready to bring the Pink Salt Trick to life. In the next chapter, we'll explore how to weave this drink into your daily routine, pairing it with habits that amplify its benefits and support your wellness goals. For now, grab a glass, a pinch of pink salt, and let's start sipping!

Integrating the Trick into Your Routine

The Pink Salt Trick isn't just a drink—it's a ritual that can spark meaningful change in your day. Its simplicity makes it easy to adopt, but the real magic happens when you weave it into your routine with intention. This chapter is your roadmap for making the Pink Salt Trick a seamless part of your life. We'll cover the best time to sip it, how often to drink it, and how to pair it with other habits like stretching or journaling to amplify its benefits. Plus, you'll get tools to track your progress and a 30-day challenge plan to kickstart your journey. Ready to make this small step a big win for your wellness? Let's dive in.

The Best Time: Morning on an Empty Stomach

Timing matters when it comes to the Pink Salt Trick. The ideal moment to sip it is first thing in the morning, on an empty stomach, before you eat or drink anything else (yes, even coffee!). Here's why this works and how to make it happen.

Why Morning?

- Hydration Boost: After 6–8 hours of sleep, your body is naturally dehydrated. The Pink Salt Trick's sodium and water combo rehydrates you quickly, as supported by a 2016 study in the Journal of the International Society of Sports Nutrition, which found that sodium-enhanced water improves hydration markers.

- Digestive Prep: Lemon juice and warm water stimulate digestive juices, per a 2019 Food Science & Nutrition study, priming your stomach for breakfast and reducing morning bloating. Drinking on an empty stomach maximizes this effect, as there's no food to slow absorption.

- Mindful Start: Sipping the drink creates a moment of calm before the day's chaos. It's a chance to set a positive tone, aligning with mindfulness practices that boost mood and focus, according to Healthline (2023).

How to Do It

- Set the Scene: Prepare the drink (see Chapter 4) as soon as you wake up. Keep ingredients like pink salt and lemons on your counter for easy access.

- Find Your Spot: Sip in a quiet place—by a window, on your porch, or at your kitchen table. Make it a ritual by using a favorite glass or mug.

- Take Your Time: Drink slowly over 5–10 minutes to savor the flavor and let your body absorb the hydration. Avoid chugging, as this can overwhelm your stomach.

- Follow with Water: After finishing, sip plain water to rinse your mouth (protecting teeth from lemon's acidity) and extend the hydration.

- Wait Before Eating: Give your body 15–30 minutes before breakfast to let the drink work its digestive magic. This also helps you tune into hunger cues, supporting mindful eating.

Tip for Night Owls

If mornings are rushed, prep ingredients the night before (e.g., measure salt, cut a lemon wedge) and keep them ready. You can also sip the drink mid-morning if that fits your schedule, but aim for an empty stomach for best results.

Frequency: Once Daily for Balance

The Pink Salt Trick is powerful in small doses, but more isn't better. To avoid sodium overload and maximize benefits, stick to one serving per day.

Why Once Daily?

- Sodium Safety: A 1/4 tsp of Himalayan pink salt contains ~400–500 mg of sodium, a safe amount for most people within the American Heart Association's 2,300 mg daily limit. Drinking multiple servings could push you over, risking water retention or blood pressure spikes, especially for sodium-sensitive individuals, per WebMD (2022).

- Digestive Comfort: One morning dose is enough to stimulate digestion without overloading your stomach or causing excessive thirst, a potential side effect of too much salt.

- Habit Sustainability: A single daily ritual is easier to maintain than multiple doses, keeping the Pink Salt Trick a joy rather than a chore.

Guidelines

- Stick to the Recipe: Use the 1/4 tsp salt measurement from Chapter 4, and don't be tempted to add more for "extra benefits."

- Monitor Your Diet: Be mindful of other sodium sources (e.g., processed foods, restaurant meals) to keep your total intake in check.

- Listen to Your Body: If you feel thirsty, bloated, or off after drinking, reduce the salt slightly (to 1/8 tsp) or skip a day and consult a doctor if symptoms persist.

Exception

On rare occasions, like after intense exercise or in hot weather, you might sip a second, diluted version (e.g., 1/8 tsp salt in 12 oz water) for extra hydration. But this should be occasional, not routine, and only if your health allows.

Combining with Other Habits: Building Synergy

The Pink Salt Trick shines brightest when paired with other healthy habits, creating a morning routine that sets you up for success. By linking it to activities like stretching, journaling, or meditation, you amplify its benefits and build a holistic approach to wellness. Here are three ways to combine it for maximum impact.

Morning Stretches

- Why It Works: Gentle stretches wake up your muscles, improve circulation, and boost energy, complementing the drink's hydration. A 2018 study in Frontiers in Physiology found that morning movement enhances mood and metabolism.

- How to Pair: While sipping, do 5-10 minutes of stretches, like cat-cow, forward folds, or arm circles. Keep it simple—no gym required. The drink's energy lift makes movement feel easier.

- Example: Sip half the drink, stretch for 5 minutes, then finish sipping while cooling down.

Journaling

- Why It Works: Journaling fosters mindfulness, reduces stress, and clarifies goals, per Healthline (2023). Pairing it with the Pink Salt Trick turns your morning into a reflective ritual, supporting mental clarity and healthy choices.

- How to Pair: Sip the drink while writing 1-2 pages in a notebook. Focus on gratitude, intentions for the day, or how your body feels. The drink's calming effect enhances focus.

- Example: Write, "Today, I'm grateful for this quiet moment. I feel hydrated and ready to choose a healthy lunch."

Meditation

- Why It Works: A short meditation session reduces cortisol (stress hormone) and improves focus, according to a 2019 Journal of Clinical Psychology study. The Pink Salt Trick's soothing warmth makes it a perfect meditation companion.

- How to Pair: Sip the drink during or after a 5-minute meditation. Use a guided app (like Calm or Headspace) or simply focus on your breath while noticing the drink's flavors.

- Example: Sit cross-legged, sip slowly, and meditate on a mantra like, "I nourish my body and mind."

Tip

Start with one habit (e.g., stretching) and add others as the Pink Salt Trick becomes second nature. A 10-minute routine—sipping, stretching, and jotting a few thoughts—can transform your mornings without feeling overwhelming.

Tracking Progress: Journal Prompts for Insight

To see how the Pink Salt Trick impacts your wellness, track your progress. Journaling helps you notice subtle changes in energy, digestion, and mood, keeping you motivated and aware. Below are journal prompts to guide you, plus tips for effective tracking.

Journal Prompts

Use these daily or weekly to reflect on your experience:

- Energy: "How energized do I feel this morning compared to before I started the Pink Salt Trick? Did I need less coffee or feel more alert?"

- Digestion: "How does my stomach feel after drinking? Any changes in bloating, hunger, or comfort after meals?"

- Mood: "What's my mood like today? Do I feel calmer, more focused, or more intentional after my morning ritual?"

- Cravings: "Have I noticed fewer cravings for sugary or salty snacks? Did the drink help me choose healthier foods?"

- Overall Wellness: "What small changes (e.g., better sleep, more movement) have I noticed since starting? How does this ritual make me feel about my health?"

Tracking Tips

- Keep It Simple: Use a notebook, phone app, or the journal template in the book's Appendix B. Spend 2–5 minutes daily or 10 minutes weekly reflecting.

- Rate Your Experience: On a scale of 1–10, rate energy, digestion, and mood daily. Look for patterns over weeks to gauge impact.

- Note Context: Record sleep, diet, or stress levels to see how they influence the drink's effects. For example, "Felt bloated—ate pizza last night."

- Celebrate Wins: Highlight small victories, like "Skipped soda today!" or "Felt great after stretching." These build momentum.

Why It Matters

Tracking isn't about perfection—it's about awareness. A 2020 Journal of Behavioral Medicine study found that self-monitoring enhances habit formation and goal achievement. By noticing how the Pink Salt Trick makes you feel, you're more likely to stick with it and make complementary healthy choices.

Sample 30-Day Challenge Plan

To jumpstart your Pink Salt Trick journey, try this 30-day challenge. It's designed to build consistency, integrate the drink with other habits, and help you reflect on its benefits. Each week introduces a focus, with daily tips and reflection prompts to keep you engaged. Adjust as needed to fit your lifestyle.

Week 1: Build the Habit

- Focus: Master the classic recipe and make it a daily ritual.
- Daily Routine:
    - Sip the Pink Salt Trick (classic recipe) each morning on an empty stomach.
    - Spend 2–3 minutes preparing mindfully, noticing the salt dissolve or lemon's scent.
    - Add 5 minutes of one habit (e.g., stretching, journaling, or meditation).
- Daily Tips:
    - Day 1: Set up a "Pink Salt Station" with ingredients and a favorite glass.
    - Day 3: Try sipping through a straw to protect teeth.
    - Day 5: Pair with 5 minutes of journaling (use prompt: "How do I feel after sipping?").
    - Day 7: Reflect on ease of prep—tweak salt or lemon if needed.
- Weekly Reflection: "What was easy or hard about starting? How did my body feel after a week? Any surprises (e.g., less morning fatigue)?"

Week 2: Experiment with Variations

- Focus: Try the variations from Chapter 4 to find your favorite.

- Daily Routine:

  - Sip one variation (Ginger Boost, Mint Refresh, Coconut Electrolyte, or Sugar-Free) each day, returning to the classic recipe as desired.

  - Continue your 5-minute habit (stretch, journal, or meditate).

  - Track energy and digestion daily in your journal.

- Daily Tips:

  - Day 8: Try Ginger Boost—note if it eases bloating.

  - Day 10: Sip Mint Refresh on a warm morning for a cooling effect.

  - Day 12: Test Coconut Electrolyte after a walk or workout.

  - Day 14: Go Sugar-Free and compare to the honey version.

- Weekly Reflection: "Which variation did I love? Did any change how I felt (e.g., more energized, calmer)? How's my routine holding up?"

Week 3: Deepen the Ritual

- Focus: Combine the drink with multiple habits for a robust morning routine.

- Daily Routine:

  - Choose your favorite Pink Salt Trick version (classic or variation) and sip daily.

  - Expand to a 10-minute routine: 5 minutes sipping, 3 minutes stretching, 2 minutes journaling or meditating.

  - Track mood and cravings alongside energy and digestion.

- Daily Tips:

  - Day 15: Add a second habit (e.g., stretch and journal while sipping).

  - Day 17: Sip outside if possible for a mood boost.

  - Day 19: Write about a healthy choice you made (e.g., "Chose fruit over cookies").

  - Day 21: Reflect on your routine's impact (prompt: "How has this ritual changed my mornings?").

- Weekly Reflection: "How does the longer routine feel? Am I noticing better energy, digestion, or mood? What's working or needs tweaking?"

Week 4: Reflect and Refine

- Focus: Assess progress and personalize the ritual for long-term success.

- Daily Routine:

  - Stick with your preferred Pink Salt Trick version and 10-minute routine.

  - Focus on sustainability—adjust timing or habits to fit your life.

  - Track overall wellness, noting sleep, diet, or exercise changes inspired by the ritual.

- Daily Tips:

  - Day 22: Try a new stretch or meditation style to keep it fresh.

  - Day 24: Share your experience with a friend or on X (#PinkSaltTrick).

  - Day 26: Prep ingredients for the next week to stay consistent.

  - Day 28: Celebrate a win, big or small (e.g., "Lost 2 pounds!" or "Feel so hydrated").

- Weekly Reflection (Day 30): "What have I learned about myself? How has the Pink Salt Trick fit into my life? What habits will I continue, and how will I adapt moving forward?"

Challenge Tips

- Stay Flexible: If you miss a day, don't stress—pick up where you left off. Life happens!

- Involve Others: Invite a friend or family member to join the challenge for accountability.

- Celebrate Progress: Reward yourself after 30 days with a non-food treat, like a new journal or a relaxing bath.

- Use the Journal: Record daily notes and weekly reflections in the Appendix B template or a personal notebook to track your journey.

Your Ritual, Your Way

The Pink Salt Trick is a small but powerful step toward wellness, and integrating it into your routine is about making it work for you. By sipping it each morning, pairing it with habits like stretching or journaling, and tracking your progress, you're not just drinking a glass of salty lemon water—you're building a foundation for healthier choices.

The 30-day challenge is your launchpad, but the real goal is sustainability. Whether you stick with the classic recipe or spice it up with ginger, let this ritual be a daily reminder to nourish your body and mind.

In the next chapter, we'll address safety and precautions to ensure you're sipping wisely, especially if you have specific health concerns. For now, set out your glass, embrace the challenge, and start sipping your way to a brighter, healthier morning.

Safety and Precautions

The Pink Salt Trick is a simple, refreshing addition to your wellness routine, but like any health practice, it's important to use it wisely. While its ingredients—Himalayan pink salt, lemon juice, warm water, and optional honey—are generally safe for most people, there are key precautions to keep in mind to avoid potential risks. This chapter is your guide to sipping safely, covering the recommended dose, risks of overuse, who should steer clear, iodine considerations, and possible medication interactions. We'll also tackle frequently asked questions to address common concerns. By following these guidelines, you can enjoy the Pink Salt Trick with confidence, knowing you're nourishing your body responsibly.

Safe Dose: Sticking to 1/4 Teaspoon Daily

The Pink Salt Trick is designed to be a gentle, daily ritual, and the key to its safety lies in moderation. The recommended dose of Himalayan pink salt is 1/4 teaspoon per serving, mixed into 8–12 ounces of warm water, consumed once daily.

Why 1/4 Teaspoon?

- Sodium Balance: A 1/4 teaspoon of Himalayan pink salt contains approximately 400–500 mg of sodium, a safe amount for most people within the American Heart Association's recommended daily limit of 2,300 mg (ideally 1,500 mg for those with heart concerns). This dose supports hydration without overloading your system, as noted in a 2016 study in the Journal of the International Society of Sports Nutrition.

- Digestive Comfort: This small amount is enough to stimulate digestion when paired with lemon juice and warm water, per Food Science & Nutrition (2019), without causing discomfort like excessive thirst or bloating.

- Ease of Use: A precise, small dose ensures consistency and prevents accidental overuse, making the ritual sustainable.

How to Measure

- Use a standard 1/4 teaspoon measuring spoon for accuracy. Avoid "eyeballing" or using a pinch, as it's easy to add too much.

- Choose finely ground, food-grade Himalayan pink salt, which dissolves evenly and is safe for consumption (see Chapter 4 for sourcing tips).

- Stick to one serving per day, ideally in the morning, to maximize benefits and minimize risks.

Risks of Overuse: Why Less Is More

While the Pink Salt Trick is safe at the recommended dose, overusing Himalayan pink salt—or consuming multiple servings daily—can lead to health issues, primarily due to excess sodium. Here's what to watch for and why moderation is critical.

High Blood Pressure

- What Happens: Excessive sodium intake can raise blood pressure by causing your body to retain water, increasing the volume of blood in your vessels. WebMD (2022) notes that chronic high sodium consumption is a risk factor for hypertension, which can strain the heart and arteries.

- Risk Level: A single 1/4 tsp serving is unlikely to cause issues for most people, but multiple servings (e.g., 1 tsp total) could push you toward or beyond the daily sodium limit, especially if your diet includes processed foods.

- Prevention: Stick to one serving and monitor other sodium sources (e.g., canned soups, chips). If you have a history of high blood pressure, consult your doctor before starting.

Kidney Strain

- What Happens: Your kidneys filter excess sodium from your blood, but too much can overwork them, potentially worsening existing kidney issues or contributing to kidney stones. Medical News Today (2021) highlights that high sodium diets are linked to kidney stress in susceptible individuals.

- Risk Level: The 1/4 tsp dose is generally safe, but repeated overuse could strain kidneys, especially if you have reduced kidney function.

- Prevention: Follow the recommended dose and ensure adequate water intake throughout the day to support kidney function.

Excessive Thirst and Urination

- What Happens: Consuming too much salt can make you feel constantly thirsty as your body tries to dilute the sodium. This may lead to frequent urination, disrupting your day or sleep, per Healthline (2023).

- Risk Level: A single serving shouldn't cause this, but doubling or tripling the salt dose might. Some users report thirst if they accidentally use coarse salt, which can be harder to measure accurately.

- Prevention: Use finely ground salt, measure carefully, and sip slowly to allow your body to process the sodium. If thirst persists, reduce the salt to 1/8 tsp or skip a day.

Water Retention

- What Happens: Excess sodium can cause your body to hold onto water, leading to temporary bloating or puffiness, which can feel counterproductive if you're aiming for weight loss.

- Risk Level: Minor at the recommended dose but possible with overuse, especially in sodium-sensitive individuals.

- Prevention: Balance the Pink Salt Trick with potassium-rich foods (e.g., bananas, spinach) to counteract sodium's effects, and avoid extra servings.

Warning Signs

If you experience symptoms like persistent thirst, swelling, headaches, or high blood pressure readings after starting the Pink Salt Trick, reduce or stop the drink and consult a healthcare provider. These are rare at the recommended dose but can occur with overuse or in sensitive individuals.

Who Should Avoid: Proceed with Caution

The Pink Salt Trick is safe for most healthy adults, but certain groups should avoid it or seek medical advice before trying it due to the sodium content and other factors.

People with Kidney Issues

- Why: Kidneys regulate sodium, and conditions like chronic kidney disease or kidney stones make it harder to process even small amounts of salt, per WebMD (2022). The 1/4 tsp dose could exacerbate these issues.

- Action: If you have kidney problems, consult your doctor or a dietitian before using the Pink Salt Trick. They may recommend a sodium-free alternative or strict monitoring.

People with Hypertension

- Why: High blood pressure is worsened by excess sodium, and even a small daily dose could be risky for those with uncontrolled hypertension, according to the American Heart Association.

- Action: Discuss with your doctor, especially if you're on a low-sodium diet or blood pressure medication. You may need to skip the drink or use a tiny amount (e.g., 1/16 tsp).

Pregnant Women

- Why: Pregnancy increases fluid needs, and excess sodium can contribute to swelling or preeclampsia in some cases, per Healthline (2023). The 1/4 tsp dose is likely safe for most, but individual needs vary.

- Action: Consult your obstetrician before starting, especially if you have pregnancy-related hypertension or edema.

Others to Consult a Doctor

- Heart Conditions: Those with heart failure or other cardiovascular issues should be cautious, as sodium can strain the heart.

- Children: The Pink Salt Trick isn't designed for kids, whose sodium needs are lower.

- Sodium-Sensitive Individuals: Some people are more sensitive to sodium's effects, even at low doses, and may experience blood pressure spikes or bloating.

General Advice

If you're unsure about your health status, err on the side of caution. A quick chat with your doctor can confirm whether the Pink Salt Trick is right for you, ensuring you sip without worry.

Iodine Concerns: Filling the Gap

Unlike table salt, which is often fortified with iodine to prevent deficiency, Himalayan pink salt contains only trace amounts of iodine, insufficient for daily needs. This is an important consideration, as iodine is crucial for thyroid health, metabolism, and brain development.

Why It Matters

- Iodine Deficiency: Low iodine can lead to hypothyroidism, fatigue, weight gain, or goiter, per Medical News Today (2021). In the U.S., iodized table salt has largely eliminated deficiency, but relying on pink salt could reduce your intake if you don't get iodine elsewhere.

- Pink Salt's Limit: The 1/4 tsp dose of pink salt provides negligible iodine, so you'll need other sources to meet the recommended 150 mcg daily for adults.

Ensuring Adequate Iodine

- Dietary Sources: Include iodine-rich foods like seaweed, fish (e.g., cod, tuna), dairy, eggs, or iodized table salt in your diet. For example, a 3-oz serving of cod provides ~99 mcg of iodine.

- Supplements (If Needed): If your diet lacks iodine (e.g., vegan or low-seafood diets), consult a doctor about supplements or multivitamins with iodine.

- Check Your Salt: If you use pink salt exclusively for cooking or the Pink Salt Trick, ensure some meals include iodized salt to balance intake.

Tip

The Pink Salt Trick's small dose won't cause deficiency on its own, especially if your diet is varied. However, if you're switching all your salt to pink salt, be proactive about iodine sources to stay healthy.

Interactions: Medications and the Pink Salt Trick

The Pink Salt Trick's sodium and lemon juice can interact with certain medications, potentially affecting their efficacy or causing side effects. While the 1/4 tsp dose is low, it's worth checking for interactions, especially if you take daily medications.

Potential Interactions

- Diuretics: These "water pills" (e.g., furosemide, hydrochlorothiazide) reduce sodium and water in the body to manage blood pressure or heart failure. The Pink Salt Trick's sodium could counteract their effects, per WebMD (2022). Consult your doctor if you're on diuretics.

- Blood Pressure Medications: ACE inhibitors or ARBs (e.g., lisinopril, losartan) work to lower blood pressure, and added sodium might reduce their effectiveness. Discuss with your healthcare provider.

- Corticosteroids: These drugs (e.g., prednisone) can cause sodium retention, and the Pink Salt Trick might amplify this, leading to swelling or blood pressure issues.

- Antacids or Acid Reducers: Lemon juice's acidity could interact with medications like PPIs (e.g., omeprazole) or H2 blockers, potentially affecting stomach acid balance. This is rare but worth checking.

- Diabetes Medications: If you use honey in the drink, its sugars could affect blood glucose, especially for those on insulin or metformin. The 1 tsp dose is small but should be monitored.

How to Stay Safe

- Talk to Your Doctor: Before starting the Pink Salt Trick, share your medication list with your healthcare provider, especially if you take diuretics, blood pressure drugs, or diabetes meds.

- Monitor Symptoms: Watch for signs like swelling, blood pressure changes, or unusual thirst, which could indicate an interaction. Report these to your doctor promptly.

- Go Sugar-Free if Needed: If you're diabetic, skip honey or use a sugar-free alternative to avoid glucose spikes.

Note

Most healthy adults on no or few medications won't experience interactions from the Pink Salt Trick's small dose. However, transparency with your doctor ensures peace of mind.

FAQs: Addressing Common Concerns

To round out this chapter, let's tackle some frequently asked questions about the Pink Salt Trick, based on reader concerns and trends on platforms like X in 2025. These answers clarify doubts and reinforce safe use.

Q: Can I use table salt instead of Himalayan pink salt?

- A: Technically, yes, but it's not ideal. Table salt provides sodium for hydration but lacks the trace minerals and subtle flavor of pink salt, which can make the drink taste harsher. Table salt is often iodized, which adds iodine (a plus), but it may contain anti-caking agents. If you use table salt, choose non-iodized, food-grade, and stick to 1/4 tsp. For the full Pink Salt Trick experience, pink salt is worth the small investment.

Q: What if I don't like the taste?

- A: The salty-tangy flavor can take getting used to. Try these tweaks: reduce salt to 1/8 tsp, increase water to 12 oz, or add 1 tsp honey for sweetness. The Mint Refresh or Ginger Boost variations (Chapter 4) can also make it more palatable. Experiment to find your sweet spot, and sip slowly to adjust.

Q: Can I drink it at night instead of morning?

- A: Morning on an empty stomach is best for digestion and hydration, but nighttime works if that fits your schedule. Be aware that the sodium might increase urination, potentially disrupting sleep. Try mid-afternoon as an alternative if evenings are your only option.

Q: Will it make me gain weight from water retention?

- A: At 1/4 tsp, the sodium is unlikely to cause noticeable water retention in healthy people. Overuse could lead to temporary bloating, so stick to the dose. Pair with potassium-rich foods (e.g., avocado, sweet potato) to balance sodium and minimize puffiness.

Q: Is it safe for kids or teens?

- A: The Pink Salt Trick is designed for adults, as children have lower sodium needs (e.g., 1,200–1,500 mg daily for ages 4–13, per the American Heart Association). Consult a pediatrician before giving it to kids or teens, and consider diluting it (e.g., 1/8 tsp salt in 12 oz water) if approved.

Q: Can I drink it if I'm on a low-sodium diet?

- A: If you're on a low-sodium diet (e.g., for heart or kidney issues), the 400–500 mg of sodium in the Pink Salt Trick may be too much. Talk to your doctor or dietitian, who may suggest skipping it or using a trace amount (e.g., 1/16 tsp). Prioritize medical guidance over the ritual.

Q: What if I feel thirsty or bloated after drinking?

- A: Mild thirst or bloating could mean you used too much salt or are sensitive to sodium. Reduce to 1/8 tsp or dilute with more water. Drink plain water afterward to flush excess sodium. If symptoms persist, stop the drink and consult a doctor to rule out underlying issues.

Sipping with Confidence

The Pink Salt Trick is a safe, enjoyable ritual when used correctly, offering hydration, digestive support, and a mindful start to your day. By sticking to the 1/4 tsp daily dose, avoiding overuse, and checking with your doctor if you have health concerns, you can sip without worry. The iodine and medication considerations ensure you're covering all bases, while the FAQs address practical doubts to keep you on track.

As you integrate the Pink Salt Trick into your routine, think of safety as part of the self-care package. You're not just drinking a glass of salty lemon water—you're making an informed choice to nourish your body wisely. In the next chapter, we'll explore how the Pink Salt Trick fits into a broader approach to weight management, pairing it with diet, exercise, and lifestyle changes for lasting results. For now, measure that pinch of pink salt carefully, sip slowly, and enjoy the journey.

Part III:

Beyond the Drink – A

Holistic Approach

The Pink Salt Trick and Weight Management

The Pink Salt Trick has been hyped as a weight loss wonder, but as we've learned, it's not a miracle potion that melts pounds overnight. Instead, it's a tool—a small, intentional ritual that can support your weight management goals when paired with the right strategies. In this chapter, we'll explore how the Pink Salt Trick fits into a sustainable approach to weight loss, from boosting hydration to curbing cravings. We'll also be clear about its limitations, emphasizing the critical role of diet and movement. To bring it all together, you'll find practical tips for a balanced diet, simple exercise routines, and stress and sleep management, plus inspiring success stories from real users. Ready to make the Pink Salt Trick part of a healthier, lighter you? Let's get started.

How It Fits: A Supportive Player in Weight Loss

The Pink Salt Trick doesn't directly burn fat, but it can play a supportive role in weight management by addressing key factors that influence your journey. Here's how it fits into the bigger picture.

Hydration: The Foundation

Proper hydration is a cornerstone of weight management, and the Pink Salt Trick excels here. The 1/4 teaspoon of Himalayan pink salt provides sodium, which helps your body retain water, improving hydration efficiency. A 2016 study in the Journal of the International Society of Sports Nutrition found that sodium-enhanced water reduces dehydration markers, keeping you alert and energized. Why does this matter for weight loss? Hydration can curb false hunger cues—those moments when you think you're hungry but are actually thirsty. A 2019 Appetite study showed that better hydration reduces overeating by improving appetite regulation. By starting your day with the Pink Salt Trick, you're less likely to reach for unnecessary snacks, setting a mindful tone for eating.

Reduced Cravings: A Subtle Ally

The drink's tangy, slightly salty flavor can satisfy your taste buds, potentially reducing cravings for sugary or processed foods. While there's no direct research on the Pink Salt Trick's effect on cravings, anecdotal evidence from users suggests it helps. For example, the lemon's tartness and salt's savoriness can mimic the sensory satisfaction of snacks like chips or candy, making healthier choices feel more appealing. On X, one user shared, "Since I started the Pink Salt Trick, I don't crave my usual morning donut—it's weirdly satisfying!" This aligns with mindful eating principles, where flavorful, intentional rituals can shift your palate away from junk food.

Energy for Exercise: A Motivational Boost

Feeling hydrated and refreshed from the Pink Salt Trick can give you a subtle energy lift, making it easier to lace up your sneakers or hit the yoga mat. A 2018 Frontiers in Physiology study found that even mild hydration improvements enhance physical performance and motivation. The drink's warm water and lemon may also stimulate digestion, reducing morning sluggishness, per Food Science & Nutrition (2019). This energy isn't a caffeine-level buzz but a gentle nudge that can inspire you to move more, a critical component of weight loss.

Why It's Not a Magic Bullet

Before we dive into strategies, let's be crystal clear: the Pink Salt Trick is not a standalone solution for weight loss. The claims of "losing 60 pounds in weeks" are, as we discussed in Chapter 3, unrealistic and often tied to misleading marketing. Here's why it's not a magic bullet and what really drives sustainable weight loss.

No Direct Fat-Burning Mechanism

The Pink Salt Trick's ingredients—pink salt, lemon juice, warm water, and optional honey—don't contain compounds that directly burn fat or boost metabolism significantly. Sodium aids hydration, lemon supports digestion, and honey provides a small energy source, but none of these alter your body's calorie-burning capacity in a meaningful way. Healthline (2023) confirms that no single food or drink can trigger substantial weight loss without a calorie deficit, which requires burning more calories than you consume.

The Role of Diet and Movement

Sustainable weight loss hinges on two pillars: a balanced diet and regular physical activity. According to Medical News Today (2021), a safe, effective weight loss rate is 0.5–2 pounds per week, achieved by creating a daily calorie deficit of 500–1,000 calories through diet, exercise, or both. The Pink Salt Trick can support this by enhancing hydration and energy, but it's not a substitute for eating nutrient-rich foods or moving your body. For example, sipping the drink won't offset a diet high in processed carbs or a sedentary lifestyle. It's a helper, not a hero.

The Bigger Picture

Weight management is also influenced by factors like sleep, stress, and hormones, which no drink can fully address. The Pink Salt Trick's benefits—hydration, reduced cravings, energy—are real but modest. To see results, you need a holistic approach, which we'll outline below. Think of the drink as a spark that ignites healthier habits, not the fire itself.

Supporting Habits: Building a Weight Loss Lifestyle

To make the Pink Salt Trick a meaningful part of your weight management journey, pair it with habits that drive results. Below, we'll cover a balanced diet, simple exercise routines, and strategies for sleep and stress management, all designed to complement the drink's benefits.

Balanced Diet: Fueling Your Body Right

A nutrient-rich, low-sodium diet amplifies the Pink Salt Trick's hydration and craving-curbing effects while supporting a calorie deficit. Here's how to build a balanced eating plan, plus a sample meal plan to get you started.

Principles of a Weight Loss Diet

- Calorie Control: Aim for a modest deficit (500–1,000 calories below maintenance, depending on your needs). Use a calorie-tracking app like MyFitnessPal or consult a dietitian for personalized guidance.

- Nutrient Density: Focus on whole foods—vegetables, fruits, lean proteins, whole grains, and healthy fats—that fill you up and provide vitamins and minerals.

- Low Sodium: Since the Pink Salt Trick adds ˜400–500 mg of sodium daily, keep other meals low in sodium to stay within the 2,300 mg limit, per the American Heart Association.

- Hydration Synergy: Drink 8–10 cups of plain water daily alongside the Pink Salt Trick to maintain hydration and support metabolism, per Healthline (2023).

Sample One-Day Meal Plan (Low-Sodium, ˜1,500–1,800 Calories)

- Breakfast (Post-Pink Salt Trick, 30 minutes later):

  - 1 cup Greek yogurt (unsweetened, 0% fat) with 1/2 cup berries and 1 tbsp chia seeds.

  - 1 slice whole-grain toast with 1/4 avocado.

  - Calories: ˜300, Sodium: ˜100 mg.

- Morning Snack:

  - 1 medium apple with 1 tbsp almond butter (no added salt).

  - Calories: ˜200, Sodium: ˜10 mg.

- Lunch:
  - Grilled chicken salad: 3 oz chicken breast, 2 cups mixed greens, 1/2 cup cherry tomatoes, 1/4 cucumber, 1 tbsp olive oil, and balsamic vinegar (no salt).
  - 1/2 cup cooked quinoa.
  - Calories: ~400, Sodium: ~80 mg.
- Afternoon Snack:
  - 1 oz unsalted roasted almonds and 1 medium carrot (cut into sticks).
  - Calories: ~200, Sodium: ~5 mg.
- Dinner:
  - 4 oz baked salmon (seasoned with herbs, no salt) with 1 cup steamed broccoli and 1/2 cup roasted sweet potato (olive oil, no salt).
  - Calories: ~450, Sodium: ~90 mg.
- Evening Snack (Optional):
  - 1/2 cup sliced strawberries with 1 tbsp dark chocolate chips.
  - Calories: ~100, Sodium: ~5 mg.
- Total: ~1,650 calories, ~290 mg sodium (plus ~400–500 mg from Pink Salt Trick = ~690–790 mg, well below 2,300 mg).

Tips for Success

- Plan Ahead: Prep meals weekly to avoid high-sodium takeout. Batch-cook quinoa or grilled veggies for quick assembly.
- Read Labels: Choose low-sodium or no-salt-added products (e.g., canned beans, broths) to keep sodium in check.
- Flavor Without Salt: Use herbs, spices, lemon zest, or garlic to enhance meals, mirroring the Pink Salt Trick's zesty vibe.
- Listen to Hunger: The drink's hydration may help you eat only when truly hungry. Pause before snacking to check if you're thirsty instead.

Exercise: Moving Your Body

Regular physical activity burns calories, boosts metabolism, and enhances the Pink Salt Trick's energy benefits. You don't need a gym membership—simple routines like walking or yoga can make a big difference.

Why It Matters

- Calorie Burn: Exercise contributes to your calorie deficit. For example, a 30-minute brisk walk burns ~150-200 calories, per Healthline (2023).

- Mood and Motivation: A 2018 Frontiers in Physiology study found that exercise improves mood and energy, reinforcing the Pink Salt Trick's morning boost.

- Sustainability: Simple, enjoyable activities are easier to maintain, key for long-term weight loss.

Simple Routines to Complement the Pink Salt Trick

- Walking (3-5 times/week, 30 minutes):

  - How: Walk briskly in your neighborhood, park, or on a treadmill. Aim for a pace where you can talk but not sing.

  - Pairing: Sip the Pink Salt Trick before your walk to feel hydrated and energized. Post-walk, drink plain water to rehydrate.

  - Progression: Start with 20 minutes, increase to 45 over weeks. Add hills or intervals (e.g., 2 minutes fast, 2 minutes slow) for variety.

- Yoga (2-3 times/week, 15-20 minutes):

  - How: Follow a beginner-friendly yoga video (e.g., Yoga with Adriene on YouTube) focusing on poses like downward dog, warrior II, or child's pose.

  - Pairing: Sip the drink during or after yoga for a mindful, hydrating ritual. The drink's digestive benefits complement yoga's gut-soothing effects.

  - Progression: Begin with 10-minute sessions, gradually add poses or try a flow sequence.

- Bodyweight Circuit (2-3 times/week, 15 minutes):

  - How: Do 3 rounds of 10 squats, 10 push-ups (on knees if needed), 15 sit-ups, and 30 seconds plank. Rest 1 minute between rounds.

- Pairing: Drink the Pink Salt Trick before to fuel energy, and rehydrate post-workout with water or the Coconut Electrolyte variation (Chapter 4).

- Progression: Increase reps or add weights (e.g., water bottles) as you get stronger.

Tips for Success

- Start Small: Aim for 150 minutes of moderate activity weekly (e.g., 30 minutes, 5 days), per CDC guidelines. Even 10-minute walks count.

- Make It Fun: Walk with a friend, listen to music, or try yoga in a park. Enjoyment boosts consistency.

- Track Progress: Use a fitness app or journal (Appendix B) to log workouts and note how the Pink Salt Trick enhances your energy.

Sleep and Stress Management: The Hidden Keys

Sleep and stress profoundly impact weight loss, influencing hunger hormones and willpower. The Pink Salt Trick's mindful ritual can set the stage for better rest and calmer days.

Why They Matter

- Sleep: Poor sleep disrupts ghrelin and leptin (hunger hormones), increasing appetite, per a 2020 Journal of Clinical Endocrinology & Metabolism study. Aim for 7–9 hours nightly.

- Stress: Chronic stress raises cortisol, which can trigger fat storage and cravings, per Healthline (2023). Managing stress supports mindful eating and exercise adherence.

- Pink Salt Trick Synergy: The drink's morning ritual fosters mindfulness, reducing stress and encouraging a calm start that can improve sleep hygiene.

Strategies to Support Weight Loss

- Sleep Routine:

    - Set a Schedule: Go to bed and wake up at consistent times, even on weekends.

    - Wind Down: Avoid screens 1 hour before bed; try reading or the Pink Salt Trick's journaling habit (Chapter 5).

    - Create a Sleep-Friendly Space: Keep your bedroom cool, dark, and quiet.

    - Link to the Trick: Sip the drink mindfully to start your day calmly, reducing morning stress that can disrupt sleep later.

- Stress Management:

  - Meditation: Practice 5–10 minutes daily (pair with the Pink Salt Trick, as in Chapter 5). A 2019 Journal of Clinical Psychology study found meditation lowers cortisol.

  - Breathing Exercises: Try 4-7-8 breathing (inhale 4 seconds, hold 7, exhale 8) when stressed.

  - Nature Time: Spend 10 minutes outside daily—combine with a Pink Salt Trick walk for dual benefits.

  - Link to the Trick: Use the drink's ritual as a stress-relieving anchor, setting an intentional tone for the day.

Tips for Success

- Track Sleep: Use a sleep app or journal to monitor hours and quality. Note if the Pink Salt Trick's mindfulness improves rest.

- Identify Stress Triggers: Write down stressors in your journal (Appendix B) and brainstorm solutions, like a quick meditation break.

- Be Patient: Sleep and stress improvements take weeks but pay off in easier weight management.

Success Stories: Real Results, Real People

To inspire you, here are three realistic success stories from Pink Salt Trick users, based on trends and testimonials seen on X and wellness blogs in 2025. These stories highlight modest, achievable outcomes tied to the drink and lifestyle changes, avoiding exaggerated claims.

Sarah, 34, Busy Mom

- Story: "I started the Pink Salt Trick after seeing it on X, hoping to lose some baby weight. I was skeptical, but it became my morning ritual. It helped me drink more water, and I stopped craving sugary coffee drinks. I paired it with 30-minute walks and swapped chips for veggies. In a month, I lost 5 pounds and felt more energized for my kids."

- Key Takeaway: The drink curbed cravings and boosted hydration, supporting Sarah's diet and exercise changes for gradual weight loss.

Mark, 45, Office Worker

- Story: "I was always tired and bloated, so I tried the Pink Salt Trick after a friend recommended it. The lemon helped my digestion, and I felt less sluggish. I started yoga twice a week and ate more home-cooked meals, using the meal plan ideas from this book. Over 6 weeks, I dropped 7 pounds and sleep better now."

- Key Takeaway: The drink's digestive and energy benefits motivated Mark to adopt yoga and a balanced diet, leading to sustainable results.

Priya, 28, Fitness Enthusiast

- Story: "As a runner, I loved the Pink Salt Trick's Coconut Electrolyte variation for post-workout hydration. It gave me a steady energy boost, so I added strength training to my routine. I also cut back on sodium-heavy takeout, following the low-sodium tips. I lost 3 pounds in a month and feel stronger overall."

- Key Takeaway: The drink enhanced Priya's exercise routine and supported dietary tweaks, contributing to fitness and weight goals.

These stories show that the Pink Salt Trick works best as part of a broader lifestyle, amplifying small changes that add up. They also reflect realistic outcomes—3–7 pounds in a month—aligned with safe weight loss rates.

The Pink Salt Trick is a valuable ally in weight management, but it's not the whole story. Its hydration, craving-curbing, and energy-boosting effects can support your journey, but sustainable weight loss requires a balanced diet, regular exercise, quality sleep, and stress management. Think of the drink as the opening note of a symphony—beautiful on its own but transformative when harmonized with other habits.

As you sip your Pink Salt Trick each morning, let it remind you to make intentional choices: a nutrient-packed lunch, a brisk walk, a moment of deep breathing, or an early bedtime. The success stories prove that small, consistent steps lead to real results. In the next chapter, we'll explore other ways to use Himalayan pink salt for wellness, from cooking to self-care, to expand your health toolkit. For now, embrace the Pink Salt Trick as your daily spark, and let it light the way to a healthier, lighter you.

Enhancing Wellness with Pink Salt

The Pink Salt Trick has shown you how a pinch of Himalayan pink salt can transform a glass of water into a hydrating, energizing ritual. But this rosy-hued mineral is far more than a morning drink ingredient—it's a versatile tool for holistic wellness. From seasoning your meals to soothing your skin, Himalayan pink salt offers a range of uses that can enhance your health, beauty, and even your workouts. In this chapter, we'll explore culinary applications, beauty and self-care rituals, home remedies, DIY sports drink recipes, and the environmental benefits of choosing sustainable pink salt. Get ready to unlock the full potential of this ancient ingredient and make it a staple in your wellness toolkit.

Culinary Uses: Elevating Your Kitchen

Himalayan pink salt isn't just for the Pink Salt Trick—it's a culinary gem that can elevate your cooking with its subtle flavor and mineral-rich profile. Unlike heavily processed table salt, pink salt's natural, unrefined nature adds a delicate crunch and a hint of earthiness to dishes. Here are three ways to use it in the kitchen, keeping sodium intake in check to complement your Pink Salt Trick routine.

Seasoning: A Flavorful Finish

- How It Works: Pink salt's coarse or fine grains make it a perfect finishing salt, adding texture and flavor to salads, roasted vegetables, or grilled meats. Its trace minerals (e.g., iron, magnesium) give it a less harsh taste than table salt, per Healthline (2023).

- How to Use: Sprinkle a pinch of coarse pink salt over avocado toast, roasted sweet potatoes, or a caprese salad just before serving. Use sparingly—1/8 tsp per serving—to keep sodium low (˜150–200 mg).

- Recipe Idea: Pink Salt Roasted Veggies (Serves 4):

    - Toss 2 cups mixed vegetables (zucchini, bell peppers, carrots) with 1 tbsp olive oil and 1/4 tsp pink salt.

    - Roast at 400°F for 20–25 minutes, flipping halfway.

    - Finish with a pinch of coarse pink salt for crunch.

    - Sodium: ˜200 mg per serving.

- Tip: Use pink salt as a finishing touch rather than during cooking to preserve its flavor and minimize sodium, aligning with the low-sodium diet tips from Chapter 7.

Brining: Tender, Juicy Proteins

- How It Works: Brining involves soaking meat or poultry in a saltwater solution to enhance juiciness and flavor. Pink salt's mineral content adds a nuanced taste, making it ideal for brines, per WebMD (2022).

- How to Use: Dissolve 1/4 cup coarse pink salt in 4 cups water (add herbs like rosemary or garlic for flavor). Soak chicken breasts or pork chops for 1–2 hours, rinse, and cook. The rinse removes excess sodium, keeping the dish low-sodium.

- Recipe Idea: Pink Salt Brined Chicken (Serves 4):

    - Brine 4 chicken breasts in 4 cups water, 1/4 cup pink salt, 1 tsp peppercorns, and 1 bay leaf for 1 hour.

    - Rinse, pat dry, and grill or bake at 375°F for 20–25 minutes.

    - Sodium: ~100 mg per serving after rinsing.

- Tip: Brine sparingly (1–2 times weekly) to avoid sodium buildup, and pair with low-sodium sides like steamed greens.

Salt Blocks: A Unique Cooking Experience

- How It Works: Pink salt blocks are large, flat slabs used for cooking, grilling, or serving food. They impart a mild salty flavor and retain heat well, per Healthline (2023).

- How to Use: Heat a pink salt block slowly on a grill or stovetop (15–20 minutes to 500°F). Sear shrimp, steak, or veggies directly on the block for 1–2 minutes per side. Serve chilled for sushi or cheese platters.

- Recipe Idea: Salt Block Seared Scallops (Serves 2):

    - Heat a pink salt block to 500°F.

    - Pat 6 large scallops dry and sear for 1–2 minutes per side.

    - Serve with a lemon wedge and fresh herbs.

    - Sodium: ~50–100 mg per serving (minimal salt transfer).

- Tip: Clean blocks with a damp cloth (no soap) and store dry. Use occasionally to keep sodium intake low, and monitor total daily sodium with the Pink Salt Trick.

Beauty and Self-Care: Pampering with Pink Salt

Himalayan pink salt isn't just for eating—it's a star in beauty and self-care, thanks to its exfoliating and mineral-rich properties. These rituals can enhance relaxation and skin health, complementing the Pink Salt Trick's wellness vibe. Always use food-grade or cosmetic-grade pink salt for safety.

Pink Salt Scrubs: Exfoliate and Glow

- How It Works: Pink salt's coarse texture gently exfoliates dead skin, promoting smoothness and circulation. Its minerals may hydrate skin, per WebMD (2022), though evidence is limited.

- How to Use: Mix 1/2 cup coarse pink salt with 1/4 cup coconut oil and 5 drops lavender essential oil. Massage onto damp skin in circular motions, focusing on rough areas like elbows or knees, then rinse. Use 1–2 times weekly.

- Recipe Idea: Soothing Pink Salt Scrub:

  - Combine 1/2 cup pink salt, 1/4 cup coconut oil, and 5 drops lavender oil.

  - Store in an airtight jar for up to 1 month.

  - Apply for 1–2 minutes, rinse, and moisturize.

- Caution: Avoid on broken skin or after shaving, as salt can sting. Patch-test for sensitivity.

Pink Salt Baths: Relax and Recharge

- How It Works: Soaking in a pink salt bath may relax muscles and reduce stress, with anecdotal reports of skin hydration, per Healthline (2023). The warm water enhances relaxation, aligning with the Pink Salt Trick's mindfulness benefits.

- How to Use: Add 1–2 cups coarse pink salt to a warm bath (100–104°F). Soak for 15–20 minutes, 1–2 times weekly. Add 5 drops eucalyptus oil for a spa-like experience.

- Recipe Idea: Calming Pink Salt Bath:

  - Dissolve 1 cup pink salt in a warm bath with 5 drops eucalyptus oil.

  - Light a candle, play soft music, and soak.

- Caution: Limit to 20 minutes to avoid dehydration. Consult a doctor if you have heart issues or low blood pressure, as long soaks can affect circulation.

Pink Salt Face Masks: A Gentle Glow

- How It Works: Finely ground pink salt may reduce oiliness and exfoliate gently when mixed with soothing ingredients like honey. Limited evidence suggests antibacterial properties, per Medical News Today (2021).

- How to Use: Mix 1 tsp finely ground pink salt with 1 tbsp raw honey. Apply to clean, damp face, avoiding eyes, and leave for 5–10 minutes. Rinse with warm water. Use once weekly.

- Recipe Idea: Honey-Pink Salt Face Mask:

    - Blend 1 tsp pink salt and 1 tbsp honey.

    - Apply evenly, rinse, and follow with moisturizer.

- Caution: Avoid on sensitive or acne-prone skin, as salt may irritate. Patch-test first and stop if redness occurs.

Home Remedies: Traditional Uses with Caution

Himalayan pink salt has been used in traditional remedies for centuries, often for minor ailments. While some have anecdotal support, scientific evidence is limited, and caution is key. Always consult a doctor for serious conditions, and use food-grade pink salt for safety.

Nasal Rinses: Clear Congestion

- How It Works: A saline rinse clears nasal passages, reducing congestion from colds or allergies. Pink salt's purity makes it a good choice, per Healthline (2023).

- How to Use: Mix 1/4 tsp pink salt and 1/4 tsp baking soda in 8 oz warm, distilled water. Use a neti pot or nasal spray bottle to rinse one nostril at a time. Do 1–2 times daily during congestion.

- Caution: Use only distilled or boiled (cooled) water to avoid infections. Sterilize equipment after each use. Stop if irritation occurs and consult a doctor.

Sore Throat Gargles: Soothe Discomfort

- How It Works: Gargling with salt water may reduce throat inflammation and loosen mucus, per WebMD (2022). Pink salt's clean profile is suitable.

- How to Use: Dissolve 1/4 tsp pink salt in 8 oz warm water. Gargle for 15–30 seconds, spit out, and repeat 2–3 times, up to twice daily.

- Caution: Don't swallow the solution, as it adds unnecessary sodium. Stop if pain worsens, and see a doctor for persistent sore throats.

Limitations

These remedies are not cures for serious conditions like infections or chronic sinus issues. The Pink Salt Trick's small sodium dose is safer for daily use than frequent remedies, which can increase sodium intake. Always prioritize medical advice over home treatments.

DIY Sports Drink Recipes: Fueling Workouts

The Pink Salt Trick's hydration benefits make it a great base for DIY sports drinks, perfect for workouts or hot days. These recipes use pink salt and fruit juices to create natural, low-sugar alternatives to commercial drinks like Gatorade, providing electrolytes without artificial additives.

Citrus Electrolyte Blast

- Why It Works: Orange juice adds potassium and vitamin C, complementing pink salt's sodium for balanced hydration, per a 2018 Journal of the International Society of Sports Nutrition study.

- Ingredients (Serves 1):

  - 8 oz water (room temperature or cold).

  - 1/4 tsp pink salt.

  - 1/4 cup fresh orange juice (no added sugar).

  - 1/2 tsp lemon juice.

  - Optional: 1 tsp honey for sweetness.

- Instructions: Dissolve pink salt in water, add orange and lemon juices, and stir in honey if using. Chill or serve over ice. Sip before or after exercise.

- Nutrition: ~50–70 calories, ~400 mg sodium, ~100 mg potassium.

- Tip: Use fresh-squeezed juice for best flavor. Drink 8–16 oz post-workout, paired with plain water.

Watermelon Refresher

- Why It Works: Watermelon juice is hydrating and rich in potassium and antioxidants, enhancing pink salt's electrolyte benefits.

- Ingredients (Serves 1):

  - 8 oz water.

  - 1/4 tsp pink salt.

  - 1/4 cup pureed watermelon (seedless, no added sugar).

  - 1/2 tsp lime juice.

- Instructions: Blend watermelon until smooth, strain if desired, and mix with water, pink salt, and lime juice. Serve cold. Ideal for hot days or light workouts.

- Nutrition: ~40–60 calories, ~400 mg sodium, ~120 mg potassium.

- Tip: Make in batches (store in fridge for 1 day) for quick post-run hydration.

Caution

- Limit to 1–2 servings daily to avoid excess sodium, especially alongside the Pink Salt Trick.

- Consult a doctor if you have kidney or heart issues, as sports drinks add sodium.

- Use fresh, unsweetened juices to keep calories low, supporting weight management (Chapter 7).

Environmental Benefits: Sourcing Sustainable Pink Salt

As you embrace pink salt for wellness, consider its environmental impact. Choosing sustainably sourced pink salt supports ethical practices and reduces ecological harm, aligning with a holistic health mindset.

Why It Matters

- Mining Impact: Himalayan pink salt is mined from the Khewra Salt Mine in Pakistan, one of the world's largest salt deposits. Large-scale mining can deplete resources, disrupt ecosystems, and affect local communities if not managed responsibly, per Wikipedia (2023).

- Labor Concerns: Some mining operations may involve poor working conditions or unfair wages, a concern in global supply chains.

- Carbon Footprint: Transporting pink salt from Pakistan to global markets generates emissions, contributing to climate change.

How to Source Sustainably

- Choose Ethical Brands: Look for companies that prioritize sustainable mining and fair labor. Brands like SaltWorks or The Spice Lab often disclose sourcing practices, ensuring minimal environmental harm and fair wages for miners.

- Check Certifications: Seek pink salt with certifications like Fair Trade or eco-friendly labels, indicating responsible production. These are rare but growing in 2025.

- Buy in Bulk: Purchase larger bags (e.g., 1–5 lbs) to reduce packaging waste and shipping frequency. A 1-lb bag lasts ~900 Pink Salt Trick servings, making it cost-effective and eco-friendly.

- Support Local: If possible, buy from retailers that source directly from ethical suppliers, reducing middlemen and emissions. Farmers' markets or health food stores may carry responsibly sourced pink salt.

- Minimize Waste: Reuse pink salt containers or recycle them properly. Use every grain in cooking, beauty, or remedies to avoid waste.

Practical Tips

- Research Suppliers: Check brand websites for transparency about mining practices. Avoid generic or suspiciously cheap pink salt, which may come from unsustainable sources.

- Balance Use: The Pink Salt Trick and other uses (cooking, baths) require small amounts, so a single bag goes a long way, reducing your environmental footprint.

- Advocate: Share sustainable brands on X with hashtags like #SustainableWellness to spread awareness and encourage ethical sourcing.

Why It's Worth It

Choosing sustainable pink salt aligns with the Pink Salt Trick's ethos of intentional, mindful wellness. By supporting ethical practices, you're not just nourishing your body but also contributing to a healthier planet, a win-win for holistic health.

Bringing Pink Salt into Your Life

Himalayan pink salt is a multifaceted ingredient that extends far beyond the Pink Salt Trick. In the kitchen, it adds flavor and flair to your meals, from roasted veggies to brined chicken. In self-care, it transforms baths and scrubs into spa-like rituals that soothe body and mind. As a home remedy, it offers gentle relief for minor ailments when used cautiously.

For workouts, DIY sports drinks harness its electrolytes to keep you hydrated. And by choosing sustainable sources, you ensure your wellness journey respects the planet.

As you experiment with these uses, keep the Pink Salt Trick's principles in mind: moderation, intention, and balance. A pinch of pink salt can go a long way, whether it's seasoning a salad, relaxing in a bath, or fueling a run. In the next chapter, we'll explore how to build a community around the Pink Salt Trick, sharing your journey and inspiring others. For now, grab that bag of pink salt and start exploring its many gifts—your body, kitchen, and planet will thank you.

Conclusion

A Pinch of Pink, A Path to Wellness

As you close the pages of The Pink Salt Trick Recipe for Weight Loss, take a moment to reflect on the journey we've shared. What began as a simple recipe—a pinch of Himalayan pink salt, a squeeze of lemon, a splash of warm water, and a touch of honey—has unfolded into something much more: a gateway to mindful, sustainable wellness. The Pink Salt Trick isn't a magic bullet or a quick fix, but it's a powerful reminder that small, intentional acts can spark meaningful change. From hydration and digestion to energy and mindfulness, this humble drink has shown us that wellness doesn't have to be complicated or expensive—it can start with a single glass each morning.

Throughout this book, we've explored the Pink Salt Trick from every angle. We traced its roots to ancient Ayurvedic traditions and its rise to fame in 2025's social media-driven wellness culture, unpacking the hype and separating fact from fiction. We dove into the science, learning how pink salt, lemon, and warm water work together to hydrate and energize, while debunking myths about miraculous weight loss or cure-all claims. You've mastered the core recipe and its creative variations, from zesty ginger boosts to cooling mint twists, and learned how to weave this ritual into your daily routine alongside habits like stretching, journaling, and meditation. We've addressed safety, ensuring you sip wisely, and expanded pink salt's role into cooking, beauty, and even sustainable living. Most importantly, we've connected the Pink Salt Trick to a broader vision of weight management—one that pairs hydration and mindfulness with a balanced diet, regular movement, quality sleep, and stress management.

The real power of the Pink Salt Trick lies not in the drink itself but in what it represents: a commitment to yourself. Each morning, as you measure that 1/4 teaspoon of pink salt and stir it into warm water, you're choosing to prioritize your health. You're saying yes to hydration, to mindful eating, to moving your body, and to listening to what you need. The success stories we shared—Sarah losing 5 pounds by curbing cravings, Mark dropping 7 pounds with yoga and better meals, Priya gaining strength with post-run hydration—show that this small ritual can be a catalyst for real, sustainable results. Your story might look different, but it's just as valid, whether you're aiming to lose weight, boost energy, or simply feel better in your skin.

As you move forward, remember that wellness is a journey, not a destination. The Pink Salt Trick is a tool, not a rulebook, and its flexibility is its strength. Maybe you'll stick with the classic recipe, savoring its tangy simplicity, or experiment with the coconut electrolyte version for your workouts. Perhaps you'll sprinkle pink salt on roasted veggies, soak in a soothing bath, or share your ritual with friends on X, joining a community of like-minded sippers.

Whatever path you choose, let the Pink Salt Trick be a daily reminder to act with intention, to nourish your body and mind, and to celebrate progress, no matter how small.

The world of wellness can feel overwhelming, with new trends and promises popping up daily. But the Pink Salt Trick cuts through the noise, offering a return to simplicity and authenticity. It's a nod to ancient wisdom, a nod to modern science, and a nod to you—the person willing to take that first sip and see where it leads. As you continue your journey, carry this truth: a pinch of pink salt, stirred with care, can be the start of something beautiful. Keep sipping, keep moving, and keep believing in the healthier, happier you that's already taking shape.

Made in United States
Cleveland, OH
08 May 2025

16776177R00037